52 WAYS TO PROTECT YOURSELF FROM CANCER

W9-BPN-755

**Terry T. Shintani, M.D., M.P.H.
and
J. M. T. Miller**

OLIVER
NELSON

THOMAS NELSON PUBLISHERS
Nashville

Copyright © 1993 by Terry T. Shintani and Janice M. T. Miller

All rights reserved. Written permission must be secured from the publisher to use or reproduce any part of this book, except for brief quotations in critical reviews or articles.

Published in Nashville, Tennessee, by Oliver-Nelson Books, a division of Thomas Nelson, Inc., Publishers, and distributed in Canada by Word Communications, Ltd., Richmond, British Columbia.

The Fat Finder's Formula is from Terry T. Shintani, M.D., *The Eat More, Weigh Less Diet*. Used by permission.

Printed in the United States of America.

Library of Congress Cataloging-in-Publication Data

Shintani, Terry T., 1951–
    52 ways to protect yourself from cancer / Terry T. Shintani and J.M.T. Miller.
        p.   cm.
    ISBN 0-8407-9672-2 (pbk.)
    1. Cancer—Prevention.   I. Miller, J. M. T. (Janice M. T.), 1944–
II. Title.   III. Title: Fifty-two ways to protect yourself from cancer.
RC268.S49   1993
616.99′405—dc20   93-7909
                                                                          CIP

1   2   3   4   5   6   —   98   97   96   95   94   93

52
· WAYS · TO ·
PROTECT
YOURSELF
FROM
CANCER

CONTENTS

GENERAL INFORMATION

NUTRITION

EXERCISE

THE ENVIRONMENTAL CONNECTION

OTHER THINGS YOU SHOULD DO

GENERAL INFORMATION

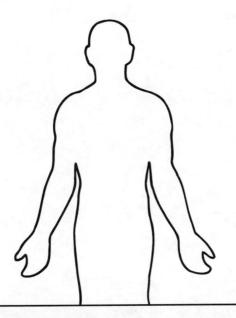

1

UNDERSTAND THE PROBLEM

The Cancer Crisis   One of every three people in the United States now gets cancer. These odds are formidable. And because this disease is now epidemic, most of us take a fatalistic attitude. We believe it's going to happen to the other guy, not us. Or if it *does* happen to us, it's just a matter of bad luck anyway, so why worry about it?

But these attitudes only amplify the epidemic because there *are* many things you can do to make certain you and those you love don't join the tragic one-third who suffer from cancer. Most of these things are simple. And if you want to learn to do everything you can to help bullet-proof yourself and your loved ones against the scourge of the twentieth century, this book is for you.

The Second Leading Cause of Death   Cancer is the second leading cause of death in Americans, right after cardiovascular disease. This year alone, according to the *U.S. Surgeon General's Report on Nutrition and Health,* more than 900,000 people will learn that they have cancer.

Some Frightening Statistics Between thirteen hundred and fifteen hundred people die from cancer every single day of the year. And the numbers are growing. If things continue as they are at present here in the U.S., some experts estimate that shortly after the year 2000 nearly 50 percent of us will be developing cancer. The possibility is staggering.

The Good News The good news is that most experts now agree that up to 80 percent of all cancers are linked to life-style and environment. That means *up to 80 percent of all cancers may be preventable!* Considering the difficulty of curing cancer once it has begun, that is good news indeed.

The Best Solution Is Prevention Despite numerous setbacks and failures, medical science is at last beginning to understand this disease. Unfortunately, advances come slowly. And many of the most common cancers—breast cancer, for example—are just as difficult to cure today as they were twenty years ago.

Some Even Better News If technology can't provide a full solution, if even the field of medicine often fails us, what can we do? The answer is *plenty!* That's what this book is all about.

The technology that will probably prevent most cancers is already in place. All we have to do is tap into it. The solution is to listen to the researchers who link diet and life-style to cancer, then create a clean environment and maximize proper nutrition. Add in the protective and curative work that the medical community is doing, and suddenly, the picture isn't quite so hopeless.

We can make an impact on the cancer epidemic right now, today. All we have to do is change our life-styles, including our nutrition and our interaction with the environment. Within a few short generations we could theoretically reverse the number of people who get cancer each year from 900,000 to 180,000—and perhaps even fewer than that. It's possible. But we're going to have to do some work. Are you ready?

2

MAKE THE MOST OF THIS BOOK

What This Book Can't Do We still have much to learn about cancer. Therefore, this book is not about incredible breakthroughs in the field of cancer research. Rather, it is an attempt to provide you with advice based on recent advances in the field of cancer prevention.

Much of this information is controversial. Thus, it is difficult to be very specific when making recommendations. In addition, each of us is unique, with unique problems. Remember this point as you evaluate the advice you find here. What works perfectly for one person may not work as well for another. For this reason, you need to work with a physician or registered dietitian before significantly altering your diet, exercise, and life-style.

What This Book *Can* Do Nevertheless, common ground in the field of cancer prevention yields simple and practical things that you can do so that you will have the best chance of preventing cancer.

The Changing Times   However, the field of cancer prevention is changing rapidly. You will be wise to make your education in cancer prevention one that continues beyond the scope and time frame of this book. In no other field of medicine is the future quite so promising as in the field of prevention of the degenerative diseases that plague humanity, including the two most common killers in America, heart disease and cancer. We *are* beginning to understand what they are, what causes them, and how to prevent them.

Use This Book Wisely   This book is designed so that you can assimilate and incorporate one new preventive measure each and every week of the year. Look at each bit of advice carefully, and discuss it with your doctor or, in the case of nutrition information, your registered dietitian (RD). Then if it is something that will apparently help you, integrate it into your life-style. If you cautiously and wisely use the information you're about to learn, you'll be able to determine what will work best for you. By doing this, you'll be taking some steps toward decreasing your risk of cancer.

3

KNOW
YOUR
ENEMY

Cell Wars   Our bodies are made up of 6 to 10 trillion cells, and each of these cells is in a constant state of change. Like miniature images of our own passage through this life, the cells are born, grow, divide, and die to be replaced by other identical cells. Some are renewed every few weeks, others take longer, but by the end of several years, it is estimated that most of the atoms in our bodies are replaced. Sometimes during this division process, changes occur to the cells, and they become malignant, or cancerous.

Cancer cells do not invade the body. They are part of the body. A malignant tumor is as much a part of you as your hair, your arm, or your heart. But it is a distorted version of you because somehow the DNA that determines how the cells will divide becomes confused. The cells lose their central blueprints and begin to reproduce at random. As the cancerous cells grow, almost all types of the various cancers produce tumors. In truth, malignant tumors are not actually dangerous unless and until they begin to seriously crowd or invade vital organs. At that point, unless something stops the progression, the individual progresses toward death.

The Four Basic Types   The word *cancer* is a catchall word for many different diseases, all of which can destroy the human body in much the same way. The basic types of cancer are the *sarcomas,* which originate in bone and soft tissues; the *carcinomas,* which originate in the tissue cells lining such body organs as the lung, colon, ovaries, breast, and skin; and the *lymphomas* and *leukemias,* which derive from the blood cells.

Understanding the Enemy   The tumors are only signs of the disease, not the disease itself. Many people make the mistake of thinking that because their cancerous tumors have been surgically removed, they are free from cancer. Often, nothing could be more untrue. If even one cancerous cell remains in the body, it can grab hold and begin the chaos anew, eventually causing all sorts of problems, including death.

Even after people have undergone surgery, chemotherapy, and/or radiation therapy, the same basic physical components that initially allowed the cell(s) to become cancerous and then allowed the body to let cancer take hold may still be in place. Cancer can quickly become a systemic disease, and it must then be treated and prevented in a systemic way. Again, that doesn't mean orthodox treatments don't work. They often do. It simply means that by thinking of cancer only as tumors, people are missing the biggest

15

part of the picture. And they need to see the big picture if they're going to win the battle.

What you do to your body today may determine whether or not you get cancer one, five, ten, or twenty years from now. The time to start preventing cancer so you never have to fight a direct battle with this disease is today, this minute.

4

UNDERSTAND YOUR IMMUNE SYSTEM

Your Defense System Chances are good that you have cancer cells floating around in your body right now. Everyone does. But chances are equally good that your natural defense system will knock the renegade cells that could cause full-on cancer out of the picture long before they have a chance to do any damage. How is that possible? Through the amazing bodily network known as the immune system.

Your immune system defends you against microbes and internal mutation. It is responsible for your very life. In fact, much of the nutritional and preventive information in this book will show you how to strengthen your immune system so the body can naturally defend itself against cancer and other disease.

Immunotherapy Unfortunately, the immune system doesn't always stop cancer cells from proliferating. Things can go wrong. But since the early

1980s, the most promising experimental treatments continue to focus on helping the immune system battle and beat cancer. The theory is that enhancing the body's immune system will be far more effective against cancer and other disease than have been the overtly invasive therapies of surgery, radiation therapy, and chemotherapy, and with far fewer side effects. Recently, researchers have come up with some amazing possibilities including a technique known as molecular surgery, which offers much hope for persons with previously untreatable brain tumors and other cancers.

How to Keep Your Immune System Strong
The most important factor in preventing cancer, though, is to keep your immune system strong enough to zap out the cancer cells before they can take hold and do you harm. There are a number of ways you can do this:

• Practice good nutrition.
• Stop smoking!
• Get regular exercise.
• Avoid physical stress.
• Avoid emotional stress.
• Watch your weight.
• Stop environmental pollution.
• Keep a positive attitude.
• Pray as often as possible.

5

KNOW YOUR AVOIDABLE RISK FACTORS

How Likely Are You to Get Cancer?   Cancer is a complex disease. It is difficult to understand, prevent, and treat in part because it is multifactorial. That is, it takes many interacting factors for the disease to develop.

If you are going to avoid being one of the 900,000 Americans who learns this year (or next) of having cancer, you need to understand not only the methods of prevention but also your personal risk. If you are at high risk, you need to take specific preventive measures.

How do you know if you're at high risk for cancer? The National Cancer Institute (NCI) offers the following guidelines.

Risks You Can Avoid

Diet   Diet is the leading cause of cancer. In 8, "Change Your Diet—Now!" you'll learn about the nutrition-cancer link. It is estimated that approximately 35 percent of all cancer could be avoided if only we'd eat right. So practice good nutrition. Often, avoiding cancer is just that simple.

Smoking   Smoking is the second largest cause of cancer. If we'd all quit smoking, most experts agree that roughly 30 percent of all cancer would be eradicated. In 9, "Stop Smoking," you'll learn exactly why smoking is such a serious health hazard.

Sunlight   Skin cancers are increasing faster than any other form of cancer in the world. The incidences of malignant melanoma, a very deadly and hard-to-treat form of skin cancer, have doubled since 1980. Almost all of these cancers are caused by excessive exposure to sunlight, so you should avoid excessive sunlight (see chapter 49, "Avoid Sunlight Exposure").

Alcohol   Drinking alcohol is a definite cancer risk, especially with regard to mouth, throat, esophageal, and liver cancer. If you smoke and drink at the same time, you're multiplying your risk. If you want to minimize your cancer risk, never drink to excess or—better yet—stop drinking alcohol altogether.

X rays   Avoid unnecessary X rays. The rays can damage the DNA, which might lead to cancer. Talk to your doctor, who will let you know just how much radiation is too much.

Industrial agents and chemicals   As you'll see in 50, "Avoid Occupational Exposures," environmental pollution is a serious and preventable cancer risk factor. To help stop the cancer epidemic, let's clean up the environment. In the meantime, avoid exposure to known carcinogens.

Hormones   The NCI points out that estrogen supplementation is a potential cancer risk. So are birth control pills. Talk to your physician about this point. If the other factors in your life indicate that you're at high risk for cancer, you may want to make some lifestyle changes before you consider any hormonal therapy or supplementation.

Sexual practices   Cervical cancer is one cancer that is definitely life-style related and, therefore, preventable. Several life-style factors are known to contribute to the high incidences of this disease, such as sexual activity with those who have themselves had multiple partners, sexual activity beginning in early teens, multiple sex partners, and other imprudent sexual activities.

6

KNOW YOUR UNAVOIDABLE RISK FACTORS

Unavoidable Risks

Genetic factors   Some people are at higher risk than others simply because of their heredity. However, that is only one factor in developing cancer. Even if other members of your family have succumbed to the disease, chances are good you can still avoid it if you take strong preventive measures.

Unavoidable radiation   The NCI points out that often children and young adults are exposed to high levels of radiation that may put them at higher than usual cancer risk, especially for thyroid cancer. Although you can't avoid it if it has already happened to you, you can certainly keep from repeating the mistake with your children.

Radon gas is an invisible, odorless gas caused by the decay of uranium deposits in certain rocks. It is another form of radiation, and the EPA estimates that it is the second-leading cause of lung cancer death, right after smoking. All American homes may have some radon. Therefore, some risk might be unavoidable. However, certain radon levels are unacceptable. Check with the EPA or local authorities to determine whether or not you're exposed to radon and what you might do about it. And it may help to always ventilate your home well.

DES   Diethylstilbestrol is a drug that was given to pregnant women to prevent miscarriages some years ago. Female children whose mothers took this drug (believed back then to be harmless) are now at higher risk of developing vaginal and cervical cancer. Again, if you were one of those unfortunate children, you can beat the odds against developing full-blown cancer by practicing the advice you'll find here about smoking, nutrition, and other anticancer measures.

If You Are at High Risk . . .

Don't despair   Even if you're at extremely high risk, you can still prevent cancer. The development of full-blown cancer requires contributing factors. Even if some of your risk factors are not preventable, the contributing factors almost always are. These factors include the avoidable risk factors listed in the previous section, as well as psychological attitude, stress levels, certain viruses, and a number of other things you'll learn about in these pages.

7

ATTAIN AND MAINTAIN YOUR IDEAL WEIGHT

Obesity and Cancer Risk   *Obesity* can be defined as "the state of having excess body fat." Some experts define *obesity* as "being 20 percent above the mean weight for height." Other experts define *obesity* as "being 20 percent above ideal body mass index (BMI)," which is weight in kilograms divided by height in centimeters squared. Studies have demonstrated that obese people have higher mortality from many diseases, including cancer, and in general have shorter life spans. The National Cancer Institute advises us to maintain a desirable weight because obesity is a risk factor in some types of cancer.

Studies indicate that obese people have higher risks of cancer of the colon, prostate, breast, uterus, cervix, gall bladder, and endometrium. Why obesity contributes to these cancers is not certain; however, obesity is associated with a high-fat diet, which is in turn associated with some cancers. In addition, excess body fat can cause an increase in sex hormones, which may in turn contribute to cancer of the sex organs, including prostate, breast, uterus, and endometrium.

Diet Advice   Eating a very low-fat diet has been demonstrated to induce weight loss, even without counting calories. Studies have shown that this can occur when you limit your fat intake to 10 to 20 percent of calories. Also, eating a high-fiber whole grain and vegetable diet will fill the stomach quickly and will induce a feeling of fullness and satisfaction that will automatically prevent overeating. Furthermore, because these foods are bulky, they must be chewed well, which also causes a feeling of satisfaction and helps curb your appetite. Some studies suggest that a diet high in complex carbohydrates (starches) tends to increase your metabolic rate slightly so that you burn calories a little faster. That makes it a little easier for you to keep your weight down. Fortunately, the recommendations here for avoiding obesity also help prevent cancer (as you'll find when you get to the nutritional advice in this book).

Exercise Benefit   Finally, don't forget the value of exercise. Regular exercise helps you burn calories while you're running, and it helps you burn calories faster even while you're resting.

8

CHANGE YOUR DIET—NOW!

The Diet Connection   In 1984, the American Cancer Society made public the first government-sanctioned anticancer dietary guidelines. Today, they and most other experts agree that there's a strong correlation between diet and cancer.

Stop Eating the SAD   The Standard American Diet has the appropriate acronym SAD. The American Cancer Society and the National Cancer Institute now state that as much as 35 percent of all cancer is diet-related (and many credible researchers put this figure as high as 70 percent). Most of what we now know about nutrition and cancer is based on cross-cultural epidemiological studies rather than on the rigorously controlled clinical studies some would prefer. Still, the epidemiological studies have proved highly valuable. They've set the stage for the more methodical studies now being conducted at research centers around the world, and the hard data are coming in. Available studies suggest that what we eat is a very large factor in determining whether we'll get cancer or be spared.

Eat Five for Fitness   On July 1, 1992, the National Institutes of Health initiated the first Five a Day Program, intended to increase public awareness of the value of eating more vegetables and fruits. The program encourages people to eat at least five, and as many as nine, servings a day of fresh fruits and vegetables. There is mounting evidence that substances in them may help prevent cancer.

9

STOP SMOKING

The Number Two Killer   Everyone now knows that smoking causes lung cancer. In fact, experts say we could do away with 30 percent of all cancer if everyone would stop smoking. Warnings by the Surgeon General have appeared on every cigarette package in the United States for years. Yet, our government refuses to prohibit the sale of cigarettes, even though taxes from tobacco sales don't begin to offset the $70 billion spent annually in health-care costs for smoking-related illnesses.

No doubt about it, smoking is a killer. Smoking also contributes to heart disease, which beats out cancer as the number one killer of all Americans. Since smoking contributes to both heart disease and cancer, it's been estimated that smoking contributes to one in five of all deaths in this country!

But since we're focusing on cancer, let's look at cancer directly caused by smoking. We all know that smoking causes lung cancer. Smoking also contributes to cancer of the oral cavity: the lips, tongue, and nasal cavity. It contributes to cancer of the larynx and the pharynx. (Cancers of the head and neck are among the absolute worst cancers to treat because of the horrible complications associated with them.) Smoking also contributes to cancer of the esophagus and bladder, and it has been implicated in cancer of the pancreas, kidney, and stomach.

What's Wrong with Smoking?   Why is smoking such a major cause of cancer? Because cigarettes are among the most noxious substances known to human beings. They are the only major American product allowed on the open market that are deadly when used as directed. One police officer who had been stricken with lung cancer made the point well in some anticancer commercials. He said that the cigarettes in his pocket were far more dangerous than the bullets in his gun. And he was right because more people die each year from lung and other smoking-related cancers than are killed by all the handguns in this country. Smoking is the leading cause of cancer deaths in men, and it has recently overtaken breast cancer as the leading cause of cancer deaths in women.

How the Killer Works   When the cigarette burns and the smoke is inhaled, it takes on a new and very dangerous character. Toxic substances that are powerful carcinogens are produced. They are found in every puff of smoke and mix in with the tar so it sticks to the lungs when inhaled. It's a wonder that even more lung cancer is not produced by such means. And of course, it sticks to everything else in the mouth and throat.

When a smoker coughs, this disgusting substance gets swallowed and even affects the stomach. The body tries to clear it out of the system by filtering it out through the kidneys, and then the kidneys and bladder are affected by this very toxic group of compounds. Studies have shown that smokers have a far greater amount of mutagens in their urine than do nonsmokers. Mutagens are things that stimulate mutation, which can cause cancer. That's enough reason to quit smoking right there.

Secondary Smoke But maybe all that doesn't matter to you. If it doesn't, consider this: smoking is known to cause cancer in those who breathe the air that smokers pollute, which is known as *secondary smoke*. Your friends, your family, and your children breathe this smoke. So to combat cancer, STOP SMOKING, AND STOP RIGHT NOW!

10

AVOID
ALCOHOL

Deadly Drink? Estimates are that approximately 3 percent of all cancers are related to alcohol consumption and approximately 2 percent of all female cancer deaths and 4 percent of all male cancer deaths are attributable to alcohol. This rate may be adjusted upward for female cancer deaths in the near future since a recent Harvard study indicates that alcohol may be a risk factor for breast cancer.

A cancer that is clearly associated with alcohol is primary liver cancer (hepatocellular carcinoma) as opposed to metastatic liver cancer that has originated at other sites. This cancer develops at a very high rate in alcoholics who have developed cirrhosis of the liver.

Direct Contact Risk of cancer is also increased in sites that come into direct contact with alcohol, such as carcinomas of the mouth, pharynx, esophagus, and larynx. If you smoke, you compound your risk. Some experts believe that up to 75 percent of all such cancers are attributable to combined smoking and drinking.

How Much Does It Take?   With regard to the link between alcohol and breast cancer, the Harvard study mentioned above indicated that women who have three to nine drinks per week have a 30 percent higher risk, and women who consume nine or more drinks per week have a 60 percent higher risk than those who do not drink.

There may also be a relationship between pancreatic, thyroid, stomach, large bowel, and rectum cancers, although these links are less certain. If you want to protect yourself against cancer, slow down on the alcohol. Or better yet, give it up altogether.

11

GET REGULAR MEDICAL CHECKUPS

Accurate Checkups Save Lives   Robert Shintani was only thirty-eight years old and the father of two young sons when some problems sent him to his doctor for a checkup. He learned he had colon cancer. He was given the necessary tests, then the appropriate surgery. The surgeons managed to remove the cancer.

And Robert Shintani didn't let cancer stop him. He went on to build the most successful window-covering business in the state of Hawaii; managed a happy, successful marriage; and reared and educated two sons, one of whom is an author of this book. Robert Shintani died at the age of seventy-seven (not from cancer): he lived almost forty years beyond his diagnosis of cancer. He became a sterling example of the good things that can happen to cancer patients if they get regular medical checkups. Because of early diagnosis, the cancer was treatable, and Robert Shintani overcame cancer in every way.

Survival   We know one thing with absolute certainty about cancer: *the earlier it's detected, the better the chance of a cure.* In fact, if caught in the very earliest stages, most cancers are curable. Often simple, localized surgery removes the small cancerous tumor before it has had a chance to spread.

The problem is with early diagnosis. Even the best physicians can miss the diagnosis of early cancers, despite their best efforts. With all cancer, there is a lengthy period of silent tumor growth, sometimes for many years, before the malignant cancer cells create a mass large enough to give the individual real problems—or large enough for physicians to detect. Signs and symptoms often mimic other common diseases. But difficult as these diagnoses can be, some physicians manage early detection and thus save lives.

Ultimately, however, you are in charge of your body. And even the remarkable physicians who can detect early stage disease can do so only if they have your body in front of them.

Visit Your Physician   Even cancers that can't be cured can almost all be treated: life can be extended, sometimes by many years. *But only if the cancer is diagnosed!* I can't say this often enough: GET REGULAR CHECKUPS FROM A COMPETENT PHYSICIAN.

Ask for guidance in this area from the Great Physician, and He will lead you to the right person—and He will guide that person in caring for you. If you do absolutely nothing else recommended in this book but this one thing, do this. It may save your life.

12

KNOW YOUR EARLY DETECTION GUIDELINES

Early Detection Is a Form of Prevention I hope I've convinced you to see your physician for regular cancer screening checkups. The *earlier cancer is detected, the more likely it can be treated and cured.* In fact, next to complete prevention, early detection of cancer is the most important factor in preventing deaths from this disease.

Your physician has a growing arsenal of screening techniques available for various types of cancer. Your physician can use such information as family history and nutritional habits to help determine whether you are or are not at high risk for certain types. There are also cancer-specific screening tests that can be done periodically to help detect cancer as early as possible.

Screening Guidelines In our efforts to fight the cancer epidemic, all of us should make good use of these screening tests. Toward that end, the National Cancer Institute has developed the following general screening guidelines for the most common cancers. You'll note that you can do some of them yourself.

Skin cancer   Examine your skin regularly and thoroughly, looking for anything unusual that might be cancer. Make sure your doctor examines your skin as part of your regular examinations.

Breast cancer   Women should learn how to give themselves monthly breast exams. In addition, they need clinical breast exams periodically. The NCI advises that after age forty, a woman should get a baseline mammogram (most communities offer them free at certain times of year), and after age fifty, she should have a mammogram every year or two. A woman who is at high risk for breast cancer should have examinations and mammograms even more frequently.

Uterine and cervical cancer   Women who are over age eighteen or who are sexually active should have annual Pap tests and pelvic examinations to screen for these types of cancer.

Colorectal cancer   Both men and women should have digital rectal examinations annually after age fifty to screen for colorectal cancer. Also, after age fifty, fecal occult blood testing should be done annually, and a sigmoidoscopy should be done every three to five years.

Testicular cancer   Men can learn how to give themselves monthly exams. Also, they should have regu-

36

lar clinical screenings and physical exams as part of overall checkups.

Prostate cancer   All males over age forty should have digital rectal exams to screen for prostate cancer. If anything suspicious is found, other more specific tests, such as the PSA, are available.

Oral cavity cancer   This screening includes a thorough examination of the interior of the mouth and the lymph nodes of the neck. If you're a smoker, you're at higher risk and should be screened more frequently.

Proposed Tests   Other cancer screening tests have been proposed.

Ovarian cancer   A new blood test called a CA-125 can be effective in detecting early stage ovarian cancer, though this test still has a lot of critics. Pelvic exams and ultrasounds should also be more frequent if one is at high risk because of life-style, diet, or family history.

Lung cancer   For smokers, elective yearly chest X rays have been recommended along with serum chemistry profiles. (But remember, your best bet is to quit smoking and automatically lower your risk.)

13

DON'T
BE AFRAID
OF SPECIAL
TESTS

Special Tests   If you are at high risk, your doctor might order other specific tests. Don't be afraid of them. Ask questions. The days when patients blindly accepted treatments and procedures are long gone. Some of the most common tests your doctor might want you to have are noted here.

Endoscopy   In this diagnostic breakthrough, a miniature telescope is inserted into various parts of the body so that the physician can look directly inside and literally see what's going on. A sigmoidoscopy and a colonoscopy are examples.

Cytological analysis   The term refers to the study of cells that have been removed from the human body. The well-known Pap smear is one form of cytological analysis that has saved thousands of lives because it detects early and therefore treatable cervical cancers.

Biopsy   The biopsy involves either cutting out a small bit of tumor or inserting a needle into the tumor and extracting a portion for analysis. Both are excellent means of detecting cancer and of discovering which type of cancer it is. Though a biopsy is often dreaded, most are relatively painless, and the results may give early warning and thus save your life.

These are only a few examples. Your physician might recommend other special tests. Be sure to ask questions about every aspect so you'll be informed and comfortable about what is being done. If you feel uncomfortable about something, you should consider getting a second opinion.

14

LEARN
YOUR
WARNING
SIGNS

Make Things Easy on Yourself   One way you can make your physician's task of early detection easier is to know the signs and symptoms of cancer. The American Cancer Society (ACS) offers the following seven key warning signs:

- Change in bowel or bladder habits
- A sore that does not heal
- Unusual bleeding or discharge
- Thickening or lump in the breast or elsewhere
- Indigestion or difficulty swallowing
- Obvious change in a wart or mole
- Nagging cough or hoarseness

The ACS is careful to advise you that many other things can also cause these symptoms, but if the problem lasts longer than two weeks, it's time to see your doctor.

Watch out for these other things:

- Chronic fatigue
- Prolonged depression
- Sudden loss of appetite
- Unexplained and chronic pain
- Any other unusual and troublesome changes in your body
- Long-term paleness
- Unexplained bruising

Take Charge   You can help prevent and/or combat cancer by being aware of your body. Participate with your physician in the task of early detection. Let her know about any suspicious signs or symptoms. Don't be afraid to report them because most of the time, they are false alarms indicating problems that are easily controlled. But do report them *early* so that if they do indicate cancer, you can catch it in time for a total cure.

15

LEARN FROM OTHERS' MISTAKES

The Melting Pot   The United States has become a melting pot of cultures and immigrants. And no matter what their cancer risks in their country of origin, almost all of these immigrants gradually fall prey to the same high incidences of cancer—and the same types of cancer—as do other Americans. This curious fact led researchers to study correlations, and this research in turn led to our first major information about the nutrition-cancer link.

Death by Fast Food and Tobacco   Scientists continue to study what happens to diverse ethnic groups when they immigrate and adopt the high-fat, low-fiber Standard American Diet. And as the world at large is dotted with American-based fast-food chains, the patterns of cancer begin to resemble those of the United States. But the fast-food chains *may* be the innocent purveyors of ill health, unaware of the problems their methods of preparing food are causing (to give them the benefit of the doubt, assuming they've been locked into their board rooms with no media for the past twenty years).

On the other hand, the American tobacco companies should know what current scientific thinking indicates as they market their product abroad in the wake of the growing resistance here in the United States. They are exporting a product that can and often does lead to death.

Searching for Causes   Much vital information has been gained through epidemiological studies about many forms of cancer, among them breast cancer. It has been one of the most studied types of cancer largely because until 1990, it was the leading cause of cancer deaths among women (it has since been topped by lung cancer). As long ago as the 1940s and 1950s, researchers began to see a high correlation between breast cancer rates and the prosperity of certain countries. In Holland, England, Denmark, Canada, Switzerland, New Zealand, and the United States, breast cancer death rates were five to seven times higher than in developing countries, such as Thailand, El Salvador, Sri Lanka, and the Philippines.

Other cancers show similar comparisons. For some twenty years now, researchers have been trying to explain the varied geographical findings. Many of their studies were conducted in Hawaii, which has a large and constantly shifting immigrant population. The results of these studies have changed the way we look at cancer and have, for the first time, given us significant and applicable information to help us prevent cancer.

43

The Fallen Victims   In the long and tedious time it has taken researchers to finally begin to get to the bottom of the problem, countless millions of people have died agonizing deaths. They had no idea why their bodies were betraying them; physicians had no idea of how to treat them.

But now we do know a great deal more about cancer. Today's tragedy is that too few of us are putting this information to good use! Even the people who claim to be eating healthier are all too often only making token accommodations to the problem, for instance, by cutting back on known carcinogens! The cancer rates continue to skyrocket, and people continue to die agonizing deaths.

We now know that smoking, poor diet, and numerous other factors cause cancer. Why can't we put this hard-won information to better use and stop some of the 80 percent or more of cancer deaths that may indeed be preventable?

16

PROTECT YOUR CHILDREN AGAINST CANCER

Stop the Epidemic—Now   Many of us suffer from cancer today because our parents unwittingly failed to protect us against it. Not that we can blame our parents. Many of their parents failed to protect them.

Even a decade ago, most people had no idea what factors contributed to cancer. The theory that diet and life-style were primary culprits had the medical establishment in an uproar for years, so how could our parents or grandparents have known?

Give Your Kids a Chance   But now we do know, and we know how to give our children the best possible chance of beating the odds against this disease. In fact, our generation could be the last one that has to do battle with cancer as an epidemic! Wouldn't that be wonderful?

Take Action   Many of us will pass or have passed along genetic predispositions to cancer to our children. Much as we regret this, nobody can change heredity. What you can do, though, is provide an environment that helps your children adopt a life-style that will likely prevent cancer and not trigger it, whether or not the genetic predisposition to the disease is a strong one. Here are some suggestions.

Stop smoking   Your smoking can give your children cancer. It also gives them the impression that it's okay for them to smoke. You may be fostering a lifelong habit that is very destructive to your children and to your grandchildren.

Don't feed your children cancer-causing foods   This book offers tips for eating foods that prevent cancer and avoiding those that promote cancer. Try to incorporate this information into your family's meals, not just your own. Most cancers take many years to develop, and the time to start preventing them is during childhood. Some studies suggest that breast cancer is initiated during childhood, and that to prevent breast cancer, altering the diet in childhood may be even more important than in adulthood. This situation may also be true for other hormone-related cancers, such as prostate cancer, ovarian cancer, and uterine cancer.

The trick in getting your children to eat right is to provide tasty, healthy alternatives to the junk food and fast foods they eat today. Make sure that cancer-preventive snacks are available; for example, fruits, oil-free popcorn, and healthy cookies. Whole grain cereals such as low-fat granolas (and *watch* that fat content) make excellent snacks.

Cut the fat   In any case, stop feeding your children fried foods, including fast foods. Many low-fat foods will provide the whole family with a nice break from meat-centered meals. They're also far easier on the pocketbook, as are almost all anticancer foods.

Offer healthy choices   Give your children healthy choices, such as good foods, alcohol-free and smoke-free environments, and options for exercise. Then let them decide. With smaller children, you'll have an easier task. But all children will learn by your example. The best thing you can do to keep from giving your children cancer is to change your life-style and diet, and let them know why!

Lead an environmentally responsible life-style   Although only a fraction of cancers (about 2 percent) are caused by pesticides and other carcinogenic environmental agents as compared to diet (35 percent by conservative estimates), this problem is getting worse. Whatever you can do to protect your environment will help.

If you do all these things, you'll be doing your best to protect your children against cancer—and you'll be helping to stop this terrible epidemic.

NUTRITION

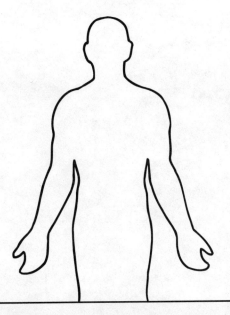

17

KNOW
YOUR
NUTRITION

Don't Dig Your Own Grave   As you've already learned, diet is a serious problem in America. In this country (and in many others), we are literally digging our graves with our knives and our forks.

Whereas the National Cancer Institute (NCI) and the American Cancer Society (ACS) attribute up to 35 percent of all cancers to poor nutrition, many experts now believe the percentage might be much higher. New reports on the nutrition-cancer link are being published every day in such prestigious medical journals as the *New England Journal of Medicine (NEJM), Lancet,* the *Journal of the American Medical Association (JAMA),* the *American Journal of Clinical Nutrition (AJCN),* and *Cancer and Nutrition (C&N).*

In 1991, John Weisburger wrote in the *American Journal of Clinical Nutrition:*

The main human cancers are associated with complex life-style-related causative, enhancing, and inhibiting factors. Tobacco smoking or chewing exposes humans to genotoxic carcinogens and to promoting substances. Likewise, Western dietary traditions involve certain carcinogens and promoters, whereas Oriental traditions implicate other carcinogens and promoters. Importantly, in virtually all situations regular intake of fruits and vegetables appreciably lowers the risk of cancer.

Lowering the Risk   The NCI has begun full-blown clinical trials so we may better understand the nutrition-cancer link. But as you've already learned, nutrition is an extremely difficult area to study. There is as yet no reliable way to determine precisely which quantities of which foods people ingest unless they are kept in a laboratory or other controlled environment for long periods of time—which is prohibitively expensive and also sometimes unethical. Plus, even in such controlled circumstances, it is still difficult if not impossible to determine which prior dietary factors and genetic predilections they brought into the environment with them. The NCI studies, like all the other studies that have recently begun, are intricate and will take years to show results.

But why wait for the results of the experiments? The recommendations made are already known to be healthy in other respects. So why not start eating right today?

18

CUT
THE
FAT

A Strong Connection According to the U.S. Department of Health and Human Services' 1984 publication *Diet, Nutrition, and Cancer Prevention,*

> The evidence is growing that eating too much fat (both saturated and unsaturated) may increase your chances of getting cancers of the colon, breast, prostate, and endometrium. Reducing fat in your diet may reduce your cancer risk. It can also help control your weight (obesity is another cancer risk factor) and can reduce your risk of heart attacks and strokes.

Fat Feeds Tumors Numerous studies (some dating all the way back to the 1940s) show that when you feed rats too much dietary fat, they often get cancer, and those that already have cancerous tumors frequently show tumor growth in direct correlation to the amounts of dietary fat intake. The National Cancer Institute's Division of Cancer Prevention and Control has approved a long-awaited study to determine the effect of dietary fat on breast and colorectal cancers and heart disease. Again, it will be years before the definite conclusions are in.

In the meantime, one of the best ways to battle cancer is to *cut back—way back—on dietary fats.* The problem is, how do we tell which foods are indeed low fat and which simply have deceptive labeling?

The solution is to use a little simple math. With the Fat Finder's Formula, you'll never again be deceived by a food label. Turn the page to find out what to do.

19

LEARN THE FAT FINDER'S FORMULA

Did You Know?   These examples make it obvious that you can't always believe what you read on food labels.

- Fat-free mayonnaise actually contains more than 37 percent fat.
- Ninety-one percent fat-free burgers are actually 49 percent fat.
- Hot dogs are 83 percent fat. (They should be called fat dogs.)

The Truth About Food Labeling   It's essential that you learn how to identify the fats in your diet if you're going to lower your risk of getting cancer and other degenerative diseases. Yet how can you do that when the fat information on food labels contains some of the greatest lies in modern marketing?

All too often, the fats in foods are hidden or skillfully disguised on the food labels—and deliberately so. For example, 2 percent fat milk is 2 percent fat by weight, not by calories. By calories (the way you should be measuring), it is actually about 35 percent fat. Whole milk is only 3.3 percent fat by weight but is actually 55 percent fat by calories.

According to recent research, the ideal anticancer, antiheart-disease diet is approximately 10 to 15 percent fat. But it's going to be impossible for you to reach this ideal without knowing how much fat is in the food you purchase, prepare, and eat.

Become a "Fat" Detective   How do you become a "fat" detective to uncover all the nefarious advertising and labeling practices that could undermine your health? This is where the Fat Finder's Formula (FFF) comes in. The Fat Finder's Formula is like Sherlock Holmes's magnifying glass. It offers you a way to look right past the apparent nutritional contents of any given product and see to the core of things. Said another way, the FFF is a calculation that allows you to determine the percentage of fat in your food.

Fighting Back with the FFF   Here's the formula. Take the grams of fat (usually found on the food label), and multiply them by nine (the number of fat calories per gram); then divide the answer by the total number of calories in the food. Your answer will give you the proportion of fat as a decimal figure. To convert it to a percentage, simply multiply by one hundred.

A good example is hot dogs, supposedly less than 30 percent fat, but they're measuring the fat by the weight of the product rather than by calories. In reality, when the hot dog is 30 percent by weight, it turns out to be 83 percent fat by calorie. And it is the percentage of fat per calories that matters, and that physicians talk about when they tell you to cut back your fat intake to 35 or 20 or even 10 percent. Even chicken hot dogs (which are often labeled as being less than 20 percent fat) are not much better. Using the FFF, you realize that chicken hot dogs are about 73 percent fat.

You'll be astonished by the amount of fat in so-called fat-free foods. Recently, I saw an advertisement for a cholesterol-free, fat-free mayonnaise. The fine print points out that there is less than one-half gram of fat per serving. They've shrewdly rounded the fat gram content down to zero. But the serving is so small, one tablespoon, that it contains only twelve calories, which means that the fat content is relatively large. If we use the FFF, we see that .5 gram times 9 calories equals 4.5 calories, and 4.5 divided by 12 equals 37.5 percent. This fat-free mayonnaise is actually 37.5 percent fat!

Work to Stop Deceptive Food Labeling

It's apparent now that too much dietary fat has severe consequences on American public health, and it's long past time that these deceptive practices were stopped. For the moment, you're on your own when it comes to detecting the fat in your food. Fortunately, the FFF allows you to calculate the deception and get to the truth.

20

USE THE FAT FINDER'S FORMULA AT THE SUPERMARKET

Tricks of the Trade   Let's take a quick stroll through the aisles of a major supermarket and look carefully at some products.

Tartar sauce   has a serving size of 1 tablespoon, which contains 5 grams of fat and is 50 calories. Using the Fat Finder's Formula, 5 grams of fat times 9 equals 45. Divide that by 50, and you get .9, which means this product is 90 percent fat! If you're trying to eat the recommended anticancer low-fat diet, stay away from this one.

Potato chips   Whole potatoes are 1 percent fat by calorie. Let's see what happens when potatoes are turned into potato chips. One serving (about ten chips) contains 7 grams of fat and 105 calories. Multiply 7 grams by 9, and you get 63. Divide that by

105, and you get .6, so potato chips are 60 percent fat. Better stay with the whole potato.

Cheese crackers (one-inch square, ten per serving) have 3 grams of fat and 50 calories. Multiply 3 grams of fat by 9, and you get 27. Divide that by 50, and you get .54. Multiply that by 100, and you have crackers with 54 percent fat.

The Bottom Line So don't trust food labels. Watch the calories, the fat by calorie, the overall fat content, and the true cholesterol content. The bottom line is, when choosing food, read the labels and use the Fat Finder's Formula. If it's fresh produce and doesn't require labeling, you're better off because fresh produce—with a few exceptions such as avocados, olives, and coconuts—is almost always low in fat.

21

EASE UP ON THE RED MEAT

Red Meat and Colon Cancer   The December 12, 1990, issue of the *New England Journal of Medicine* (*NEJM*) published a study showing that women who eat beef, lamb, or pork on a daily basis may have a 2.5 times higher risk of colon cancer than those who eat little or no red meat. Since colon cancer is the third leading cause of cancer death (right behind lung and breast cancers), this finding may be an important confirmation of what many nutritionists have believed for some time.

About 110,000 new cases of colon cancer will be diagnosed this year. Some 60,000 people will die from it. The *NEJM* study confirmed that many of these deaths could be prevented because one key reason for this tragedy is a high-fat, meat-centered diet. What diet can cause, diet can probably prevent.

The American Meat Lobby Naturally, the spokespeople for the American meat industry are up in arms, arguing that meat is essential to human nutrition. And I suspect that the concept won't sit too well with a lot of other people, either, especially not with those of us who believe that there is something inherently American about eating good, red meat. But in the past twenty to thirty years, hormones, antibiotics, and other chemicals have been extensively used by the meat industry to "doctor" up the meat they produce. When we eat meat, we can't avoid eating the residues of all these unnatural substances. The *NEJM* study provided evidence that dietary fat *isn't* the only carcinogenic substance in red meats. (Nor is it the only one in other foods.)

Red Meat and Other Cancers Apparently, the red meat connection doesn't stop with colon cancer. Red meats and their fats are also strongly linked to the incidences of breast, uterine, and prostate cancer, and evidence is mounting that the list includes even more types of cancer.

Takeshi Hirayama of the National Cancer Research Institute in Tokyo has monitored 122,000 people for decades. His conclusion is that "those who consume meat daily face an almost four times as great risk of getting breast cancer as those who eat little or no meat." A growing number of other researchers concur. So watch your red meat consumption. It may help save your life.

22

EASE UP
ON THE
POULTRY

Poultry One of America's favorite foods is fried chicken. We've already talked about what fats can do to the human body. Now let's talk about the chicken.

The Modern Bird Most contemporary anti-cancer literature advises people to substitute chicken and fish for red meats. How good is this advice?

Although it's true that chicken and fish have fewer fats than does red meat, poultry still has plenty of fat —even without the frying. Turkey is somewhat better than chicken but not much. Other birds—ducks and Cornish game hens—have even more fat than does chicken. Whichever kind of bird you eat, you're going to get more fat than you need. (It does help to take off the skin, but do this *before* you cook, or the fat is already cooked into the poultry.)

But there are even worse problems with the modern bird. The most serious ones are discussed here.

Birds, like cows, pigs, and sheep, are made from animal protein. Many experts believe that there is a correlation between intake of animal protein and many solid cancers.

In addition, salmonellosis has become a serious problem. This occurs in part because of new resistance to antibiotics caused by overuse intended to counter the unsanitary and unwholesome conditions in which some chickens and other poultry are reared. Poultry can also be dosed with toxic chemicals (in the feed, mostly as pesticides and herbicides) and artificial hormones. These substances are associated with increased risks of cancer. Next time you're hungry for a fried chicken, consider all this, and consider easing up on the poultry.

23

EASE UP
ON THE
FISH

Fish   Contemporary experts tell us that eating fish is a good bet—especially cold-water fatty fish—because they are rich in the Omega-3 fatty acids believed to decrease risks of heart disease and also inflammation caused by autoimmune diseases. However, there is a possibility that when you eat the fish, you may also be getting more than you bargained for.

PCBs   The April 1992 issue of the *Archives of Environmental Health* published a study headed by Dr. Frank Falck. It suggested that PCBs (pesticides) cause breast cancer. The evidence was strong enough to encourage the NCI to begin full-scale studies, starting in 1994. The published study, done at Hartford Hospital in Connecticut, found that the fatty breast tissue of women with breast cancer contained more than twice as many PCBs and DDEs (another pesticide) as did comparable tissue from non-cancerous breasts.

America's water is heavily polluted with pesticides. Because fish breathe the water they swim in, they are especially vulnerable to contaminants in the water. Because the bigger fish eat the smaller fish, by the time we eat the bigger fish the level of toxicity may be quite high. Scientists have also found data suggesting that PCBs may be tumor promoters in such cancers as malignant melanoma.

And though we are often reassured that PCB levels are generally lower than the governmental tolerance level, nevertheless, the cancerous breast tissue studied by Dr. Falck's group discovered PCBs about a thousand times higher than the safety guidelines of the Food and Drug Administration. Gives you something to think about, doesn't it?

Do You Have to Give Up Everything? By now, you must be thinking that you'll have to quit eating altogether. Not at all. There are still plenty of delicious foods you not only can eat but should eat. But to stop this cancer epidemic (as well as the heart disease, diabetes, and all other diet-related degenerative disease plaguing this country), we're all going to have to make some serious changes in our eating habits. For example, various studies show that vegetarians tend to live longer and have lower rates of heart disease and most major forms of cancer.

Meat, Birds, and Fish as Condiments If you must have fish, start using it as a complement to your meal rather than as your main dish. This approach can also work with red meat and poultry. Asians have been particularly savvy about this technique for centuries (or were until they began to adopt the Standard American Diet). Many of their traditional dishes are vegetable centered and merely flavored with small amounts of meat, and they're delicious. Not only is it a healthier way to eat, you'll never believe how much you can save on your food bills until you try it.

24

KNOW YOUR DAIRY PRODUCTS

The Protein Connection People once believed that dairy foods were essential to human health because they contained a great deal of protein and calcium. The idea of the importance of protein, though scientific in basis, was quickly overdone, for it became the foundation of an advertising ploy by the dairy and meat industries. But we now know that animal sources may be *too* high in protein for human good. High protein diets block the reabsorption of calcium in our kidneys and cause it to leak away in our urine. In addition, high animal protein diets are associated with certain cancers. Therefore, eating too much protein is ill-advised.

Perfect Food? Dairy food is also very high in fat and cholesterol. Besides these factors (which increase the risk of many types of cancer as well as heart disease), dairy food is probably the single largest cause of allergy in children and adults, though it is seldom detected.

Recently, a study done in Norway found a close correlation between the consumption of dairy food in various countries and the incidence of juvenile onset diabetes. In addition, the American Pediatrics Association now recommends that whole cow's milk not be used for infants under nine months because it can cause anemia.

Lactose   Another problem with dairy food is that it contains lactose. Lactose is a form of sugar found in milk. We digest it easily as children, but as we become adults, most of us lose the ability to digest it. This suggests that adult human beings were not originally designed to eat dairy food.

The Calcium Connection   Calcium has long been the primary reason for the recommendation of dairy food as an "essential" food. The reason for this emphasis is the concern over osteoporosis, a disease that causes bones to break easily and backs to hunch over with age. Lack of dietary calcium certainly contributes to osteoporosis, but it is important to recognize that many factors contribute to osteoporosis, such as lack of exercise, excessive protein intake, estrogen imbalance, lack of vitamin D, smoking, and other life-style factors.

In addition, it is important to recognize that there are excellent sources of calcium other than milk that have no cholesterol, are low in fat, are not excessive in protein, and have more calcium per calorie. Dark, leafy greens are a good example. Although one cup of milk contains 244 mg of calcium, it has 150 calories. Compare that to one spear of broccoli, which contains

205 mg of calcium and 50 calories, one cup of collard greens, which has 148 mg of calcium and only 25 calories, and one cup of turnip greens, which contains 197 mg of calcium and only 30 calories. Another type of green that is an excellent source of calcium is seaweed. One cup of kelp contains 317 mg of calcium and only 60 calories. There are many types of seaweed that can be prepared deliciously, such as in Japanese dishes. In fact, dulce was eaten plain by the Irish people for many, many years.

Poor John   The next time you drive or drop by a Baskin-Robbins ice-cream store, think about poor John. He is the self-exiled son of the Robbins side of the equation, and he walked away from his family fortune because he didn't like where the money came from. He has written *Diet for a New America,* and what he has to say about dairy food might give you nightmares.

He states that the amount of toxic substances used today in dairy farming has grown from a trickle to a torrent. He cites the effects of growth hormones and other modern animal husbandry techniques on dairy food. Cattle are kept in such unhealthy conditions that sickness becomes epidemic. They are shot up with antibiotics, drugged, dosed with growth hormones, and sedated for milking.

Back to Basics   Maybe dairy food as God designed it wasn't all that bad for us, though there is much debate about how much of even that we were expected to consume. But dairy food as human beings have *redesigned* it is a concoction that we could well do without. Especially if we want to do everything possible to combat cancer—and win!

25

GIVE UP REFINED SUGAR

Know Your Carbohydrates   Carbohydrates come in different forms. Simple carbohydrates are also known as sugars. Complex carbohydrates are better known as starches.

Some people worry about eating starches because of the long-standing myth that starches cause you to gain a lot of weight fast. But calorie for calorie, starch calories are less fattening than fat or oil calories. Biochemical studies show that for starch to be converted to body fat, about 23 percent of the calories in the starch is burned in the conversion process. Only 77 percent of the calories can show up on your waist or hips. Fats or oils burn only 3 percent of their calories while processing the fatty acids that your body needs directly for nourishment. That leaves 97 percent of the calories available to be converted to "love handles."

In fact, one component of starchy food that can

help people lose weight is the dietary fiber. Dietary fiber is the nondigestible part of foods. It may help prevent some types of cancer. But make sure you're eating your starches in an unrefined form so they are high in fiber. For example, eat brown rather than white rice, brown rather than white bread. Eating whole foods such as vegetables or whole grains provides enough dietary fiber so that you feel full and you actually find yourself losing weight in addition to getting healthier and doing all you can to prevent cancer. Dietary fiber also slows the absorption of calories so that you stay satisfied longer.

No More Candy Bars   Though there is no direct link between white and other refined sugars and cancer, there is an abundance of evidence that refined sugar is generally bad for your overall health. Probably the worst thing about refined sugar is that it is the source of empty calories. That is, it has no anti-cancer nutrients or fiber in it, and the danger is that it replaces foods that do. The foods to stay away from include white sugar, brown sugar, candy bars, and all other sugary products (watch those cereals!). These devitalized foods provide nothing but calories.

Substitutes   But you don't have to give up all sweets just because you give up refined sugar. Fresh or dried fruits will quickly satisfy your sweet tooth. You'll get used to the taste of these whole food substitutes and will soon find you're eating better than ever!

26

KNOW YOUR FREE RADICALS

Free Radicals   We've known for decades that there is no *one* cause of cancer. Rather, cancer comes about as a result of a number of variables, all interacting to set the stage for the mutated cells to grow uncontrolled in your body.

In the process of this cellular rebellion, standing head and shoulders above the enemy swarm of cancer triggers and promoters are certain cancer-causing substances known as free radicals. These little insurgents are the by-product of normal metabolic activity, and the size of their invading force depends almost entirely upon you because certain of the most lethal types of them can swim right in as part of what you eat—or *don't* eat.

DNA   The microscopic code for our very existence is kept in the DNA of each cell in our bodies. The DNA dictates what type of cell each cell will be and determines when the cell will grow and when it will stop growing. These basic units of matter are further made up from atoms, which are composed of protons and electrons spinning around a center, or nucleus. Free radicals are atoms containing an extra unpaired electron that can spin free and collide with other molecules, thus damaging the cell membrane and disturbing the DNA. This damage can be the first step to cancer, heart disease, inflammatory problems, and perhaps more than fifty other diseases and physical problems.

Oxidation   Free radicals can be caused by many things, both internal and external. They are formed by a process known as oxidation. The rust on your car and the discoloration and spoilage of your food result from oxidation, that is, the oxygen molecules reacting with the molecules of the given substance. The process of oxidation actually releases energy in the form of highly dangerous and volatile oxygen radicals (free radicals). Free radicals can also be caused by ultraviolet light (perhaps accounting for the growing incidences of skin cancer) and by other forms of radiation. And whereas the body's natural defenses can usually block and tame any free radical attack, the free radicals run out of control if the body's defense system is down.

Free Radical Scavengers   Enter the Good Guys. Free radical scavengers are also known as antioxidants, and they are crucial to the prevention of cancer. They intercept the free radicals, bond to the unpaired electron, and neutralize it so it can't harm your DNA.

Where do we find these Good Guys? In many vitamins, minerals, and other micronutrients. Therefore, many of the anticancer nutrients are known as anti-oxidants. Among this white-hatted army are the vitamins A, C, and E; the minerals selenium and zinc; and other nutrients, some known, some yet to be discovered.

27

KNOW YOUR ANTICANCER VITAMINS

What Vitamins Can Do Evidence is growing that vitamins can protect us against certain cancers. But there is still controversy in this research. Of the thirteen organic substances that scientists have identified and labeled as being vitamins, only a few have even been examined with regard to their potential in the war against cancer.

Mounting Evidence for Prevention Nevertheless, there *is* hard-to-ignore evidence of causal links between good nutrition and the *prevention* of cancer, and it appears that the immune system plays a strong role in the battle against cancer. Most experts have no trouble admitting that vitamins and minerals and other micronutrients definitely play a key role in keeping the immune system in fighting shape.

A lot of very good people are doing some very good

work and are coming up with evidence that certain vitamins may be critical in preventing many types of cancers. In the next few chapters, you'll learn about some of this work. Whether or not you choose to follow the advice is up to you and your physician.

How to Get Your Vitamins   Should you get your vitamins in natural foods or as a supplement? Frankly, whole foods are always far better weapons against all disease than are derived parts, vitamins included. In fact, most of the studies correlating vitamins with lowered cancer risk are done with whole foods rather than with vitamin pills. So vitamins, if possible, should ideally be eaten in their natural state, which means as part of a whole food. And ideally, our foods will be pure and fresh enough to deliver all the nourishment we need if only we eat right.

28

KNOW YOUR BETA-CAROTENE

A Curious Correlation   As we've seen, smoking causes cancer—about 30 percent of all cancers in the United States. And yet some people can apparently smoke and not get lung cancer, while others are almost guaranteed to get it. Which raises a question that has puzzled scientists for years: Why do some people get certain kinds of cancer, while others who live almost identical life-styles don't?

Again, the preliminary answers to the puzzle have come through epidemiological, or ethnic, studies. In Hawaii, for instance, the native Hawaiian population has the highest rate of lung cancer, followed by Caucasians. Japanese, Chinese, and Filipino males who smoke the same amount have far fewer cases of cancer. What makes the difference?

Cancer Protection   Researchers' best guess so far is that it's not genes that protect some ethnic groups and not others, but nutrients in their diets. Smokers who eat a large amount of high beta-carotene foods are apparently at lower risk of getting cancer than are smokers who don't eat these foods. Feed the others the same amounts of these healthy foods, and you'd likely get similarly low cancer statistics. And of course, people who don't smoke at all have an even lower risk of getting lung cancer. There is also evidence that beta-carotene helps prevent many other forms of cancer.

Where to Get It   Foods high in beta-carotene include carrots, mangoes, papayas, cantaloupes, squash, pumpkins, oranges, broccoli, asparagus, and other dark green, red, and yellow fruits and vegetables. The recommended intake varies from person to person, but you won't go wrong if you eat it in its natural state and go for several high beta-carotene vegetables and fruits every day. And remember, as with all foods, it's better to get your nutrition from its natural state if possible.

Beta-carotene is a powerful nutrient. In fact, clinical trials are being held to study its effectiveness in the possible treatment of cancer. You don't have to wait for the trial results. Start eating right *today*.

...side note here. In 1943, ...Ernst Krebs and his... granted a patent for a synthetic substance they called pangemic acid, or vitamin B_{15}. It was also called Krebiozen. They claimed it had miraculous properties and could provide relief from asthma, arthritis, cancerous cell proliferation, and so on. Beware! Experts say there is no such vitamin. In fact, when investigators analyzed the contents of various bottles labeled B_{15}, they found differing substances. The bottles so-labeled contain anything the manufacturer chooses to put in them. They haven't been proven safe, and they haven't been proven effective. Nobody can even yet prove what's in the various bottles!

Vitamin B_{17}   In the early 1950s, Ernst Krebs also helped introduce laetrile to the U.S. Another "false" vitamin, this invention stirred up an equal or greater amount of controversy as did Krebiozen. The main problem was that the compound contained potentially lethal amounts of a precursor to cyanide, and an even slight overdose could prove fatal. Hundreds of reports and studies have been done on the effectiveness of laetrile as a cancer treatment, and several Mexican clinics still make it their cancer therapy of choice.

However, in well-controlled trials, laetrile was shown to be no more effective than a placebo. Even those who claim it works admit it works only when the patient is on a vegetarian diet. Which brings up the issue of whether laetrile ever had any effect at all.

30

KNOW YOUR VITAMIN C

Miracle at Vale of Leven   Linus Pauling won the Nobel Prize for chemistry in 1954, then won the Nobel Peace Prize in 1962. So people paid attention when, in 1979, he published a study called *Vitamin C and Cancer*. In it he offered up the results of a trial he'd done with advanced cancer patients at Vale of Leven Hospital, Loch Lomondside, Scotland. He had used megadoses (ten grams per day) of vitamin C to bring a 4.2-fold increase in survival time for one group of dying patients as compared to matched controls.

The medical community was both skeptical and hopeful. If the tests could be duplicated, vitamin C might be at least a component of a miracle cure. Pauling did more testing, then concluded that "the ingestion of large amounts of vitamin C is of definite value in the treatment of patients with advanced cancer . . . and has even greater value for the treatment of cancer patients with the disease in earlier stages and also for the prevention of cancer." However, these studies and conclusions were later refuted by well-controlled trials at the Mayo Clinic.

The Current Claims   But over the years, evidence has shown that though vitamin C may not cure cancer, it may be protective against cancers of the esophagus, larynx, oral cavity, pancreas, stomach, rectum, breast, lung, bladder, and cervix. There may be others as well.

Today, the National Cancer Institute, the American Cancer Society, the National Academy of Sciences, the National Institutes of Health, and physicians all over the world will tell you to eat your anticancer fruits and vegetables—especially ones that contain high amounts of vitamin C. This vitamin is yet another antioxidant and may combat cancer on several levels at once. In addition to direct free radical action, it may boost the immune system and protect in that way. It may help to eliminate carcinogens such as nitrosamines. And it may also strengthen the body's tissues.

Where to Find It   Vitamin C can be found in ample amounts in oranges, lemons, limes, avocados, the cruciferous vegetables, spinach, asparagus, peas, tomatoes, and many other tasty foods. To determine the amount of vitamin C you need to eat and/or take as supplements, you'll need to do further reading and consult your physician or registered dietitian.

31

KNOW
YOUR
VITAMIN E

Another Cancer Fighter   Fewer studies have been done on vitamin E (chemically known as tocopherol) than on the other two antioxidant vitamins, A and C. Nevertheless, a growing body of evidence suggests that vitamin E is also a cancer fighter.

Boosting the Immune System   Like many other anticancer nutrients, vitamin E is most effective in its role of enhancing the immune system. However, studies at New York Medical College have shown vitamins A and E to be effective against fibrocystic breast disease, which in rare instances may turn into breast cancer. This may possibly be seen as an indirect anticancer benefit.

Other Benefits   Researchers published a study in *Nutrition and Cancer* describing how they fed mice vitamin E after chemically inducing cancer.

They found a decreased incidence and rate of tumor growth as compared to a control group that was not fed vitamin E supplements. Another study noted in *Nutrition and Cancer* examined the role of vitamin E as protection against environmental carcinogens and concluded that it was effective. Vitamin E has also been shown to positively affect cellular enzymatic activity, one place where breakdown might lead to cancer.

Don't Overdo It   However, the first study also showed that when the dosage of the vitamin E was increased tenfold, the benefits vanished. The same principle may hold true with other nutrients. There is a point of critical mass beyond which you may be doing more harm than good.

So—how much is too much? Unfortunately, there's no hard-and-fast answer. Individual differences, differences in eating habits and in environment, make it impossible to prescribe for anyone without a physician's consultation. Use the RDA as your guideline. If you're really considering serious dietary change, see your physician or registered dietitian.

If you just follow the National Institutes of Health's advice about eating at least five to nine helpings of fresh fruits and vegetables every day, you'll go a long way toward getting all the good nutrition you need (barring special problems). Here is more specific advice:

- Eat at least one vitamin A–rich selection every day.
- Eat at least one vitamin C–rich selection every day.
- Eat at least one high-fiber selection every day.

- Eat cabbage family (cruciferous) vegetables several times each week.

The nutritious foods that contain vitamin E include dark green leafy vegetables, whole grains, walnuts, almonds, and peanuts, among others.

32

AVOID NITRITE-CURED, SMOKED, AND PICKLED FOODS

Esophageal Cancer Esophageal cancer is the sixth most common cancer in the world and an especially difficult type to treat. The May 30, 1992, issue of *Lancet* published a study by K. K. Cheng et al., conducted in Hong Kong, that correlated the Chinese epidemic of esophageal cancer with drinking soups and/or drinks at high temperatures, infrequently consuming leafy green vegetables and citrus fruits, smoking tobacco, drinking alcohol, and getting a high intake of pickled vegetables. It was the first case control study to show an association between pickled vegetable consumption and esophageal cancer risk. The study strengthens other evidence of the carcinogenicity of the N-nitroso compounds.

Stomach Cancer Researchers have long known that there is a high correlation between the nitrates and nitrites (N-nitroso compounds) and cancer of the stomach. And whereas stomach cancer has decreased in the U.S. (from the leading cause of cancer death in the first half of the twentieth century to the eighth today), it is still a major cause of cancer death in Japan and other Asian countries.

The geographical variations of the disease have led to epidemiological (regional/ethnic) studies, which have long shown that people whose diets are high in smoked, salted, barbecued, and pickled foods are at greatest risk. Japanese people who immigrate to the United States and adopt the SAD find a tenfold drop in stomach cancer risk after just two generations. Unfortunately, with the decreased risk of stomach cancer comes an increased risk of the types of cancers killing other Americans—lung, breast, colon, and prostate.

Say No to Nitrates and Nitrites   Nitrates and nitrites occur naturally in various foods such as beets, radishes, celery, and spinach but do not represent a problem in and of themselves in these vegetables because balancing nutrients are also part of the foods. But these N-nitroso compounds are also found —without the countereffect and in higher proportions—in smoked and pickled foods and may also be heavily used as food preservatives. And here, they can mate with the amines in your stomach to form highly carcinogenic compounds called nitrosamines. Nitrosamine-producing foods include hot dogs, bologna, most lunch meats, sausages, bacon, and any smoked or pickled meat.

Say No to Anthracenes   Just as when you smoke tobacco, when you barbecue or smoke foods, toxic substances are produced. The difference is, they go straight to the stomach so the digestive organs get the full cancer-causing effect. Anthracenes, found in ordinary barbecue smoke, are especially mutagenic and can lead to cancer. You can also get in trouble with them if you grill things too long.

33

AVOID MOLDS

Foods That Cause Cancer   Are there foods that should never be eaten, foods that can directly cause cancer?

You bet there are! In fact, many molds and fungi have been shown to cause experimental cancer. Two dangerous types are mycotoxins and toxic mushrooms. Since most poisonous mushrooms will simply kill us outright, we don't have to worry about them causing cancer. But the aflatoxins? That's another problem altogether. Aflatoxin is a specific mycotoxin produced by Aspergillus flavus, which is the most potent cancer-producing substance ever discovered. Tests with animals have led us to detect a direct relationship between the aflatoxin levels in food and rates of liver cancer in England, Africa, China, and Southeast Asia.

The problem is not just with the foods but with freshness because these molds and fungi develop only in nuts, grains, seeds, and rice that become stale and moldy.

Foods to Watch Out For   Some food products that could develop aflatoxins when moldy include the following:

- Peanuts and peanut butter
- Pecans, pistachios, and almonds
- Cornmeal and grits
- Cottonseed meal

If these are fresh, most make excellent additions to your diet. But if they're moldy, beware. In addition, there are other cancer correlations with nonfresh foods. Always watch out for spoilage or rancidity in *all* food.

34

KNOW
YOUR
SOYBEANS

Healthy Hogs One possible anticancer food that most Americans are missing out on is the lowly soybean. This food has been a staple in Asia for centuries, but in the United States, it's been processed into oil and used to make margarine or mayonnaise or other things that are especially bad for you. Or it's been used to make protein meal for hog feed. We've had some very healthy hogs here in the United States—not so many healthy people.

Soybeans Whole soybeans are high in vitamin A, calcium, phosphorus, and iron. They can be boiled and eaten whole, sprouted and eaten whole, fermented and turned into soups, or processed into nutritional flours and grits. They are also now processed into texturized vegetable protein, or TVP, a tasty meat substitute that can be simulated to taste like ham, beef, bacon, or any other meat product and can be used in any way that meat can.

In Japan, soybeans have been turned into tofu and miso soup. Soybeans may be an anticancer nutrient. Some experts believe that the lower incidences of breast cancer among women in Japan is in large part attributable to their high intake of soybeans (and also seaweed). And though gastric cancer is still the number one killer in Japan, a study by Takeshi Hirayama published in *Cancer and Nutrition* indicates that soybean paste soup (miso) may lower the incidence of even that.

Protease Inhibitors   Some possible anticancer components of soybeans have been isolated. They are known as protease inhibitors and flavonoids. They are also found in chick-peas and lima beans and a few other plants and seeds, and they may be tumor-blocking substances.

A High-Fat Food   On the other side of the coin, soybeans are also high in fat. They are roughly 40 percent fat by calories. Tofu, a popular soybean product, is roughly 50 percent fat. As you know, high-fat diets are associated with obesity and with some cancers. So know your soybeans and enjoy them, but be careful not to overdo it when you add them to your diet.

35

EAT YOUR CRUCIFEROUS VEGETABLES

Healing Flowers When viewed from the top, the flowers of the cruciferous family of vegetables form a cross. That is how they get their name. And these little vegetables apparently help ward off cancer.

Sulforaphane Recently, Dr. Paul Talalay of Johns Hopkins University headed a research team that discovered a tumor-blocking chemical called *sulforaphane*. It exists in broccoli, brussels sprouts, cauliflower, kale, carrots, and green onions.

Indoles In other experiments, substances called *indoles* were isolated from cruciferous vegetables, then added to the diets of mice who had experimentally induced lung and stomach cancers. The indoles clearly stopped the tumor growth. There is great hope that either or both of these substances (sulforaphanes and indoles) may make up the cancer drugs of the future.

Prevention Is Better Than Cure   However, we can already use sulforaphanes and indoles to prevent cancer so that we never have to go through the difficulties of treatment. We can eat them directly.

Perhaps that is why cruciferous vegetables have been linked to reduced risk of cancer of the colon, lung, esophagus, larynx, rectum, prostate, and bladder. And most members of this family are high in vitamin A, vitamin C, and the mineral selenium, all of which have been linked to reduced cancer risk. Other isolated substances may also do direct battle with certain kinds of cancer.

What They Are   The cruciferous family includes broccoli, brussels sprouts, cabbage, cauliflower, bok choy (a Chinese cabbage), collards, horseradish, kale, kohlrabi, mustard greens, radishes, rutabagas, turnips (don't forget the greens), and watercress.

36

EAT
PLENTY
OF FIBER

The Fiber Factor   Fiber is the indigestible part of vegetables, fruits, and whole grains. Both the National Cancer Institute and the American Cancer Society recommend a high-fiber diet for the prevention of colon cancer. Years ago, Dr. Denis Burkitt observed low rates of colon cancer in areas of Africa where consumption of fiber was high. In fact, industrial nations where dietary fiber intake is low have rates of colon cancer up to eight times higher than those of developing nations where dietary fiber intake is high.

There's also an apparent link between too little dietary fiber and other conditions, such as diverticular disease, irritable bowel syndrome, and diabetes. Unfortunately, not all that many of us have taken this information to heart—or to the dinner table. Colon cancer is still the second most common form of cancer. A full 5 percent of the U.S. population—men and women alike—will develop this disease.

Fiber and Colon Cancer   Some experts believe that dietary fiber helps prevent colon cancer by increasing the bulk of the stool and thus increasing transit time and decreasing the time that the colon walls may be exposed to any carcinogenic substances that may be found in the stool. Fiber may also help prevent cancer by binding carcinogenic substances and rendering them less active, or by altering the colonic flora, which may also play a part in producing carcinogenic substances.

Fiber and Breast Cancer   The *Journal of the National Cancer Institute* (April 3, 1991) published a study indicating a possible link between dietary fiber and breast cancer. Laboratory rats fed twice the amount of fiber commonly found in our Western diets developed many fewer breast tumors than did the test rats who received little or no fiber. In fact, the results were similar to laboratory findings for studies comparing low-fat to high-fat diets.

How Much Is Enough?   The National Cancer Institute tells us that Americans now eat about eleven grams of fiber daily. It recommends that this amount be increased to about twenty to thirty grams daily, not to exceed thirty-five grams daily because of possible adverse side effects. Any number of health-enhancing foods contain such high amounts of fiber. Bran is best, though legumes (beans of various kinds) are right up there. But we can also get ample amounts of fiber from cruciferous vegetables (broccoli, cauliflower, cabbage, brussels sprouts, turnips, spinach, and rutabagas); other vegetables (carrots, celery, asparagus, etc.); fruits (blackberries, apples, peaches, raisins, etc.); as well as beans, seeds, and all types of whole grains.

Watch Out for Fiber Fraud   Be careful when buying cereals, breads, and other fiber products. For a food to qualify as fiber rich, it should contain four or five grams per ounce. A good rule of thumb is to avoid preprocessed foods altogether. Stick to good old oatmeal and other whole grain cereals and un-processed fruits and vegetables. In other words, stick to whole foods, and you won't go wrong.

37

EAT FRESH FRUITS AND VEGETABLES

Spoilage Fruits and vegetables can begin to spoil the moment they are picked—and sometimes even before. Spoilage means that bacteria attack the substance of the food and break it down through enzymatic activity.

We try to slow down this decay in several ways. We freeze, refrigerate, can, dry, blanch, dehydrate, spice, sugar, and chemicalize our foods. Sometimes foods are processed into lifeless pulp, then we try to revitalize them by adding processed forms of the nutrients we eliminated. And unfortunately, as we do all these things to prevent spoilage, we reduce nutritional content so that soon we're no longer eating much real food at all.

Without the nutritional content in food, we're loading our bodies with calories to process—and we're not even kind enough to provide the nutrients necessary to protect ourselves.

The Example of Vitamin C   When trying to decide if eating fresh food is worth the small amount of extra time and energy you'd have to invest, consider these few facts about food and vitamin C taken from Arnold E. Bender's *Food Processing and Nutrition:*

- Lima beans lose 48 percent of their vitamin C after forty-eight hours at room temperature, and 70 percent after ninety-six hours.
- Lettuce and broccoli stored in a wire basket in a refrigerator for three days lose 30 percent of their vitamin C.
- Steaming causes a loss of 15 to 20 percent of the vitamin C in kohlrabi, brussels sprouts, cauliflower, and potatoes.

Buy Fresh, Eat Fresh   Although most nutrients don't degenerate this fast, it's still best to buy your food as fresh as possible, as close to its natural state as possible, and prepare it as quickly as possible after you've purchased it. That way, you'll be getting the absolute best from your food.

38

LEARN ABOUT JUICING

The Newest Diet Fad Everywhere you look, people are selling juicers and books about juicers, and they are talking about juicing. They make claims from the sublime (weight loss) to the ridiculous (near-eternal life). What is this thing about juicing?

The Nutrition Fresh fruit and vegetable juices are delicious, compact ways to ingest megadoses of vital nutrients. There's nothing wrong with that. But juice is not a whole food; it is processed through a juicer. Any nonwhole food can present problems if consumed in vast quantities over prolonged periods of time.

Fiber As you've seen, fiber is essential to human health. When you juice foods, you're squeezing most of the fiber out. Even if you get plenty of fiber in other parts of your diet, it's probably not wise to throw away the fibrous parts of vegetables and fruits all the time. Whole foods are perfect foods, designed just as God wanted them to be. (And after all, His wish for us is perfect health.) When you throw away the fibrous part of the food, you may well be throwing away some of the little understood micronutrients that prevent cancer, too. We just don't know enough about food and the way it interacts with the human body yet to take such risks.

Sweet Juices   Some juices, especially fruit and carrot juices, are high in sugar. Drinking large volumes of them over prolonged periods of time can have an adverse effect on your system, causing wide swings in your blood sugar levels.

Healthy Sources   So much for the bad news. The good news is that fresh vegetable and fruit juices are some of the richest sources of vitamins, minerals, and enzymes available to humanity. If you don't overdo it, adding them to your daily diet can be one of the best things you've ever done for yourself.

The Truth About Processed Juices   Juices are good for you—but only fresh juices. Most commercially processed juices are essentially sugar water with colors and flavors added—and perhaps they contain a small amount of real juice. They may sit on warehouse shelves, often for months, losing most of whatever nutrients they might have had. They may also develop free radicals.

Pesticides   Unless you're fortunate enough to be able to buy organic produce, you need to be aware that the fruits and vegetables you're juicing may have been treated with pesticides and herbicides. So if you're going to do any juicing, scrub your produce well. But remember that it's still best to get most of your nutrients from the whole food.

39

KNOW YOUR ANTICANCER MINERALS

A Pill a Day?   Is it possible for a person to have a healthy diet based on a daily vitamin and mineral pill with maybe a burger or other junk food? The answer is an absolute, "No!"

Nutritional science is not advanced enough to fully analyze foods, and we don't yet understand—or even know about—many nutrients. But we do know that pills of any kind should *never* replace genuine foods.

Don't Tamper with Nature   You might get along quite well for a time on a meganutrient pill a day plus a few bowls of brown rice (or whatever), only to learn a few years down the road that you've increased your probability of getting cancer.

Vitamin and mineral pills are designed as supplements, not replacements. And they are uniformly designed after foods that are essential nutrients. Get more information before you decide to use supplements. Make sure you take the proper dosages. Talk it over with your physician.

The Cancer Fighters   Some of the anticancer minerals are also antioxidants, and so far as we know they work in much the same way as do the anticancer vitamins: that is, by acting as free radical scavengers and intercepting radical electrons. Other minerals act on the body in different ways but are still linked to cancer prevention. Altogether, the cast of Good Guys includes the following:

- *Selenium.* This potent antioxidant protects cell membranes from free radicals, among other things.
- *Calcium.* Some studies indicate that this mineral helps prevent colon cancer, among its other advantages.
- *Zinc.* This mineral's role may be indirect, but it certainly helps keep the immune system strong.

Other minerals are also vital to overall good health and may help prevent cancer in that they keep the potential victim generally strong. They include iron, phosphorous, chloride, magnesium, potassium, sulfur, and sodium. Trace minerals (of which we need only minute amounts) include selenium (see above), arsenic, chromium, cobalt, copper, fluoride, nickel, manganese, boron, and vanadium.

Though research into the role of minerals in preventing and/or causing cancer is far behind that of vitamins, the evidence is mounting that minerals, in the correct amounts, can go a long way toward helping you prevent and battle all degenerative disease, including cancer.

40

KNOW SOME PROMISING NUTRIENTS

A Nutritional "Whole" in One   We've already talked about vitamins and minerals, so here we'll talk about the other micronutrients. Some of them we understand quite well. Others remain a mystery. But scientists are feverishly trying to unravel the rest of the mystery of micronutrition because some micronutrients may well be key factors in finally solving the larger puzzle of how to best prevent and/ or treat cancer as well as other degenerative disease. Many of these chemical substances are beginning to yield their secrets. A few examples of the more recently discovered benefits of various micronutrients are included here.

Sulforaphane   can be found in broccoli, brussels sprouts, cauliflower, kale, carrots, and green onions. This chemical apparently blocks tumor formation in animals. There's strong hope it may do the same for humans (and may already be doing so since the foods it comes from have proven in numerous tests to be anticancer).

3-n-butyl phthalide is found in celery, which seems to be another anticancer food. This substance appears to lower blood pressure and reduce blood cholesterol in rats and probably has other benefits as yet to be discovered.

Chlorophyll is the substance that makes fruits, vegetables, and other growing things green. A great deal of research done with regard to its benefits as an anticancer nutrient has had mixed results.

Carotenes are the pigments that make fruits and vegetables red or orange. One carotene, beta-carotene, has already shown substantial promise as a cancer fighter. A sister substance, alpha-carotene, is under study, and scientists are enthusiastic about the expected results. Other pigments—anthocyanins (red-blue), proanthocyanidins (colorless), and flavonoids (colorless or yellow)—offer hope as disease fighters.

The "Whole" Truth These substances are only a few of what promises to be a vast range of micronutrients that fight disease. If you consistently eat processed foods, you may lose many of these beneficial nutrients, including some we don't know about yet.

That doesn't mean you should *never* eat processed food. There may be a place for that in your diet (though a much, much smaller place) as long as you have the good sense to eat whole foods most of the time.

41

EAT
WHOLE
GRAINS

The Germ of the Wheat   At some point in history, someone decided that both rice and wheat products could be improved upon by polishing the grain. White rice and white breads became symbols of status, whereas the coarser whole grain products were eaten by the "unfortunate." The irony is, of course, that the "unfortunate" people were actually fortunate in terms of their health.

The U.S. is certainly one of the wealthiest nations in history. Thanks to mass production, everyone in this country has been able to afford white bread for decades, making this altered food a staple. Chances are, you grew up eating white bread and bologna or white bread and butter. Chances are better than 35 percent, too, that you're going to get cancer unless you break your addiction to the Standard American Diet and replace it with a commonsense diet.

White vs. Whole   In the 1980s, after the fiber studies had won over the hearts of medical scientists, similar studies showed that whole grains possessed similar cholesterol-controlling abilities because they contain a significant amount of both soluble and insoluble fiber. But when you mill, or refine, grains, you strip away most of their cholesterol-fighting ability. So ease up on the white bread, the white rice, everything refined and tampered with.

Whole Foods   It's time to make the point that God created our foods to fit our bodies. All the nutritional components of any whole food are made to perfectly complement each other and to interact with perfect symmetry to nourish our bodies. Take away any one component, and you've ruined the balance that is the basis for perfect health.

According to James Mount in his book *The Food and Health of Western Man,* refining wheat flour to a 70 percent extraction rate (common) costs you high percentages of fiber, vitamin E, pyridoxine, thiamine, biotin, nicotinic acid, folic acid, riboflavin, pantothenic acid, manganese, magnesium, phosphorus, potassium, iron, and also the trace elements lithium, boron, copper, and cobalt. Who knows what other combinations of possible anticancer nutrients are left on the factory floor?

The Staff of Life   Whole grains were the central part of the diet of all the great civilizations, including the ancient Israelites, Egyptians, and Asians. Wild grains abounded in the world in biblical times, and the Middle East was the breadbasket of Western civilization. Biblical peoples ate meat during festivals, and they sacrificed meat to God in the temple. Most of the rest of the time, they ate exactly as you should be eating: whole grains, beans, vegetables, and fruits.

Types of Whole Grains   The disappearance of whole grains from dinner tables is one factor that contributes to modern degenerative diseases, including cancer. For example, in the U.S., from 1900 to 1980, the consumption of wheat decreased 41 percent, and corn 84 percent. In an attempt to reverse this trend, the National Cancer Institute advises us to "eat foods with adequate starch and fiber . . . by eating more fruits, vegetables, potatoes, *whole grain breads and cereal,* and dried peas and beans."

Because of a renewed emphasis on health in these United States, a variety of whole grains will be available to you at either the supermarket or the health food store. They will include brown rice, wild rice, millet, buckwheat, bulgur wheat, amaranth, quinoa, oats, and barley. Any vegetarian cookbook will offer you a wealth of delicious recipes showing you how to integrate whole grain dishes into your menu. In addition, a growing number of more conventional cookbooks specialize in whole grain cooking and baking. Try some of these recipes, and you'll never again be satisfied with the bland taste of white bread or overprocessed cereal grains.

42

BE A
SMART
SHOPPER

Your Goal   You'll want to do a number of things if you're going to change from a cancer-promoting diet to an anticancer diet. You'll want to

- avoid fried foods.
- avoid animal foods that inherently contain a lot of fat.
- integrate the many anticancer foods into your diet.
- limit your overall fat intake (animal *and* vegetable) to 10 to 20 percent of your overall calorie intake.
- watch out for hidden fats by using the Fat Finder's Formula.

Begin good nutrition in the supermarket. Learning to shop wisely is the first step toward cancer prevention.

Purchase Some Implements   As your budget permits, purchase kitchen implements that will help you prepare healthy foods. Buy a juicer. Fresh vegetable and fruit juices are valuable for staying healthy, although they should not replace whole foods. A good juicer will cost from $150 to $300.

A vegetable steamer will be helpful in preparing your vegetables and other tasty dishes. You can purchase one from $20 to $60.

A food processor will help you deal with the large volume of vegetables and fruits you'll be eating by reducing preparation time. It is also excellent for making your own baby foods and has a thousand other uses. Your $50 or so will be well spent.

A grater will be useful for slicing vegetables and otherwise preparing food. If you don't already own one, buy one made of stainless steel at well under $10.

A food blender is great for making shakes, smoothies, soups, and hundreds of other tasty foods. You'll spend somewhere from $50 to $250 for a good one.

Buy a stainless steel pressure cooker. Beans, grains, and vegetables cook much faster in a pressure cooker. You will save time and preserve nutrients, too. You'll spend about $50 to $100 for a good one.

Select Your Food   Stock up on an ample supply of whole grains. You might also want to buy a recipe book teaching you how to prepare delicious whole grain dishes. Make them, instead of meats, the center of your anticancer diet.

Fresh produce is especially important in an anticancer diet. The fresher the better, since some nutrients deteriorate on the shelf. You should eat as much as you want, at least five servings a day. If at all possible, buy organic vegetables and fruits. If you can't, don't be overly concerned. The cholesterol in all animal foods and the fats in many foods are far more dangerous than the pesticides that you might find on some produce.

Choose a variety of whole foods. Be adventuresome and try foods that you have never tried before. And don't be discouraged. No matter where you live, you'll be surprised at the variety of vegetables available to you once you step beyond the conventional potatoes, tomatoes, corn, and beans that you grew up with. Stay away from canned vegetables as much as possible, by the way. The best is fresh, then frozen.

The advice given about vegetables is also true for fruits. Go for variety, and try lots of recipes.

Try to eliminate most or all meats, poultry, and fish for at least one week. If you can do it, your taste sensitivities will change, and you'll find your fruits, vegetables, and grains even tastier. Most Americans are addicted to fats, salt, and sugar. These substances jade your taste buds and make other foods seem bland. If you eliminate them from your diet, the healthy foods aren't bland at all. You'll even learn a whole variety of delicious tastes that you may have never experienced before. If you have to have that meat flavor or texture, try some of the meat substitutes in your local health food store.

Choose whole foods over processed foods. Remember, our Maker designed our bodies, and He designed our foods. You'll do best if you select foods that are as close as possible to the original design.

Watch out for sugared cereals. When possible, make your own from whole grains like oats or cornmeal. Barring that, read the labels carefully. Cereals make a lot of promises on the labels that simply don't hold up to closer scrutiny.

Read the labels on *all* products. Several governmental agencies are trying to standardize labels on foods so they won't be misleading (e.g., what does "natural" mean?). But thus far, it's let the buyer beware!

Check out some of the other stores in your community, such as health food stores, open markets, and ethnic markets, if you can't find the foods you want at your local supermarket. You may be surprised at the exotic variety and the bargains you can find.

43

DON'T BELIEVE FOOD LABEL FABLES

The Food Police   For decades, some food manufacturers have gotten away with blatant deception. Fortunately, a number of medical and nutritional studies slowly but surely enlightened the public. A new wave of resistance against such deceptive practices caused the Food and Drug Administration (FDA) to finally begin enforcing regulations against false food labeling.

Now food manufacturers are protesting as the FDA seizes shipments of deceptively labeled food and otherwise forces compliance to the new ruling principle that *food consumers have a basic right to know what they're really eating.* No more bright, bold "no cholesterol" labels on plant oils and products that never contained cholesterol to begin with (but will be converted to cholesterol, labels or no, once inside the body). And now when a product says "low fat," it is supposed to mean just that. "Fresh" juices will have to be fresh, and if a bottle says "grape juice," someday soon it will actually contain more than a small percentage from the grape and a whole lot of apple juice, water, flavoring, and refined sugar.

The NLEA   A new law that will put even more muscle into the enforcement of labeling and advertising laws is called the Nutritional Labeling and Education Act. It should be in full force sometime in 1994. This bill will force all manufacturers to state, clearly and concisely, what is really in their foods. This bill will include fresh produce, and there is increasing pressure on the U.S. Department of Agriculture, which regulates meat and poultry, to adopt a similar policy.

Some companies are already beginning voluntary compliance with the new law. Others are ducking and dodging and double-talking themselves to death, trying to keep up the old subterfuge.

44

BE
A SMART
COOK

Be a Healthy Chef   You've learned the basics about nutrition, and you've learned to shop wisely. Next, you can learn a new way of preparing your foods so you won't undo all your other efforts.

Don't Pour Grease Down Your Throat   The first thing you need to learn about food preparation is that you must quit pouring grease down your and your family's throats. We Americans have somehow gotten used to the taste of fat. We live on fried foods. It's time to find alternatives.

Make Your Kitchen a Health Center   There are many things you need to start doing to cook as wisely as possible. Here are a few to get you started.

Cut out fried foods   Bake, boil, or steam your foods instead of frying them. If you must fry, learn to use a small amount of water instead of oil to keep your food from sticking to the pan. (This is called water sautéing.) If you must use oil, use the smallest amount possible, such as a small amount of spray-on oil. Use low-sodium soy or other sauces to enhance the flavors of these foods if you find them too bland without the fats.

Cut out the oil-based salad dressings   If you prepare a healthy salad, then slather it with oil-based salad dressing, you're kidding yourself. French dressing is 84 percent fat, ranch is 93 percent fat, bleu cheese is 91 percent fat, and italian is 91 percent fat. If you must eat your salads with dressing, use no-oil or low-oil dressings. Or you can make your own from blended vegetables and other low-fat products, adding spices to taste.

Slow down on the cheese sauce   Some people suggest that we enhance the flavor of broccoli by deluging it with cheese sauce. If you follow this suggestion, you'll succeed in making a healthy food far less healthy. Most of the standard cheese sauces range from 66 to 75 percent fat. The good news is, delicious and healthy sauces are available if you'll take the time to learn how to make them.

Stay away from barbecue   As you learned in an earlier section, barbecued, smoked, pickled, and nitrite-cured foods are linked to cancer. You should avoid cured foods such as bologna and give up the tempting tidbits from the barbecue pit.

Get rid of your fats, butter, oils, and mayonnaise   It will be a good deal easier for you to eliminate fats

117

from your diet if they're not even in your kitchen. You can find alternatives that will soon be just as tasty. You can use fat-free dressings and sauces, zesty salsas, fresh lemon or lime juice, or tasty spices to flavor your foods.

Keep healthy snacks on hand   Try eating fresh fruits, vegetable sticks, low-fat whole grain cookies and crackers, air-popped popcorn, and bean dips instead of candy, high-fat cookies, or other foods that are bad for you. Snacking can be good for you if you do it right.

EXERCISE

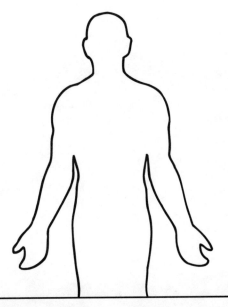

45

GET REGULAR EXERCISE

Ruth Heidrich When Ruth Heidrich was diagnosed with breast cancer, she was concerned that she'd never again be able to run and enjoy life. After her surgery, the first thing she tried to do was exercise and get back in shape. Needless to say, that was a little premature. But on the third day, she was out jogging despite the pain.

She was determined. She soon was able to again run a marathon, and she made her goal—the Ironman Triathlon. Just to do it would represent a victory over her disease because she was literally racing for her life. And she exercised and succeeded in racing herself right into several world championships in her age group. In addition to a rigorous exercise regimen, she adopted a low-fat vegetarian diet. Ten years after the initial diagnosis and surgery, she's still winning races, and she's apparently winning her battle against cancer!

Obesity and Cancer   Does exercise prevent cancer? The literature on this is not completely clear, but there is ample evidence that exercise can help prevent obesity and is an important part of any weight loss and maintenance program. And we do know that obesity correlates to various cancers, including breast, endometrial, and gall bladder cancers.

In addition, some cancers, such as breast cancer, are hormone related, and we also know that an increase in obesity causes an increase in female hormone levels. Thus, exercise may have a role in preventing cancer by helping to prevent obesity.

In both cancer and heart patients, the death rate is apparently higher among those who are either unable or unwilling to get adequate physical exercise. Furthermore, the better your physical fitness in general, the better your chances of combating any disease.

A Harvard Study   A study conducted by Dr. Rose E. Frisch of the Harvard School of Public Health has shown that women who get little or no exercise are two and a half times more likely to get cancers of the uterus, cervix, ovary, and vagina than are those who are more active. So take a tip from Ruth Heidrich. Exercise. (Be sure to check with your doctor before you start, however.) Then begin running your race for life *before* you get cancer. It will be a much easier race to win.

46

TRY WALKING

Learning to Walk   The simple act of walking may help save your life. Even though inventions all around you indulge you and encourage you to be sedentary, walking is one of the best things you can do for yourself.

You can, of course, wear your regular shoes and go for a stroll around the neighborhood every now and again. Or you can turn your walking into a full-on sport, complete with special shoes, gear, specific times of day, and other routines that will help you structure your walking into a serious activity. But if you decide to do this, you should do and know a few things.

- See your physician if you have any health problems before you engage in any exercise, and discuss what is an appropriate level of exercise for you.

- If you're over forty and haven't been getting much exercise or if you've ever had heart trouble, see your doctor before beginning a vigorous walking program.
- Buy yourself a decent professional pair of walking shoes. A mile or so into your program, you'll be glad you did.
- Invest in other clothing that will make your walks pleasant and comfortable, for instance, a lightweight jacket that will keep you warm if the wind comes up or a pair of loose-fitting slacks or shorts.
- Plan to walk thirty to sixty minutes at least every other day. Start slow, though, perhaps fifteen minutes a day for a week or so, then gradually build up.
- Vary your walking route for maximum pleasure.
- Don't forget to warm up and cool down. Several good books on walking are available at most bookstores. One of them will teach you how.

47

TRY SWIMMING

Wonderful Exercise   If you don't already know how to swim, you're missing out on a wonderful exercise. Take the time; make the effort to learn.

If you already know how to swim but don't have access to a pool or other swimming facility or area, you'll have to relegate your exercise schedule to the things that are practical. But if you do swim and can find a place to indulge yourself, you'll be able to engage in a great form of aerobic exercise.

One advantage of swimming as an exercise is that it eliminates the strain on joints and bones that can occur from prolonged walking. People who suffer from arthritis or other joint problems can indulge to their hearts' content. Again, the ideal schedule for maximum aerobic toning and conditioning is twenty to thirty minutes several times a week.

Pleasurable Exercise   As with any new exercise program, if you have health problems, be sure to check with your physician to see how much exercise is appropriate for you.

Check out your local YWCA or YMCA. It offers a number of swimming programs for all ages: underwater exercise programs for seniors, advanced swimming classes for children and teens, and nearly every water sport you can think of.

If you swim alone but in a safe place, buy a waterproof Walkman so you can listen to music. It's fun to practice water ballet on your own.

Marry your swimming program to another form of exercise, for instance, to walking. Go for a refreshing swim after a long, satisfying walk.

Take lessons. No matter how well you swim, you can doubtless improve. New strokes and new ways to use your body will make you feel a sense of achievement that can only enhance the wonderful new you who is developing as you proceed with your exercise program.

48

TRY DANCING

Where to Dance   Okay, so you're not a social animal and you don't plan to start spending your nights in ballrooms. No matter. The best kind of dancing exercise is the kind you do at home, usually in front of the TV. You can do aerobic dancing, otherwise simply known as aerobic exercise, and you have a hundred or more tapes to choose from, all the way from the several Jane Fonda tapes to Richard Simmons' party for people who love oldies.

Social Dancing   If you enjoy dancing, but you aren't eager to go to country clubs, you have another alternative. You can join an aerobic dance class. Many are open to both men and women, which means you can take your spouse or perhaps even meet one there. Or you can even start your own class. You get a dancing workout, while at the same time you have the social pleasures of doing your dancing with others.

Dancing Pointers   However you decide to do your dancing, a few pointers might help you get maximum pleasure from your new activity.

Again, if you have health problems, check with your physician.

Invest in some special clothing and/or gear. It will make you feel special.

Join a nonaerobic dance class. There are ballet classes and jazz and other modern dance classes in most communities for all age groups and all degrees of excellence. Even if you don't plan to set your hat for Broadway, dancing can be fun and give you a deep sense of accomplishment.

Design your dancing so you can work out to your favorite type of music. Aerobics tapes run the gamut from spiritual to hard rock. Choosing your favorite will maximize your pleasure.

Take it seriously. Even when you're alone, working out to a tape, give it your best. You'll get a better workout, and you'll also feel better about yourself.

Don't forget to warm up and cool down. Most videotapes and audiotapes work these stages into the program. But if you're working out on your own, remember that these two parts of the workout are vital to keeping your body working right.

THE
ENVIRONMENTAL
CONNECTION

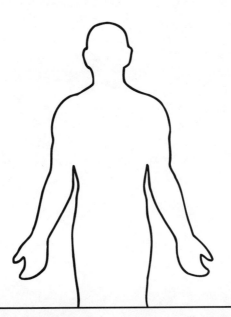

49

AVOID EXCESSIVE SUNLIGHT EXPOSURE

Common Skin Cancer   It has been estimated that about 3 percent of all cancers are related to excessive sunlight exposure. Sunlight is clearly a cause of squamous cell carcinoma and basal cell carcinoma of the skin, the two most common types of skin cancers. These cancers occur on parts of the body exposed to sunlight, and the risk of these cancers increases with the amount of exposure to the sun.

Light-skinned individuals seem to be at higher risk of getting these cancers. Melanin skin pigment may have a protective effect, since light-skinned people have lower concentrations of this pigment, and dark-skinned people, who get far fewer skin cancers, have higher concentrations of this pigment.

Malignant Melanoma   This less common but more deadly type of skin cancer is increasing faster than any other form of cancer in the world; incidences have doubled since 1980. And though the small molelike tumors can be removed if they're caught early enough, if the malignancy has spread, there is no treatment and—thus far—no cure.

The possible link with sunlight is not so clearly established as in the more common forms of skin cancer. But melanomas could be caused by excessive exposure to the sun, and it is still prudent to avoid excessive sunlight. Binge tanners and other outdoor types are most vulnerable to all types of skin cancer, especially if they have fair skin.

The American Cancer Society tells us that people who have had three or more sunburns before the age of twenty have five times the risk of getting melanoma. And this problem has probably been compounded by the depletion of the ozone layer in our atmosphere. The ozone layer shields us from harmful ultraviolet radiation. As it is depleted, the ultraviolet rays beam down on us more intensely than they would otherwise, perhaps making the risk of skin cancer even higher.

The ozone layer is vanishing at a frightening rate —all because of environmental pollutants. Learn what you need to know to stop its destruction, and you'll reduce the risk of melanomas and other skin cancers and help to save future generations of people from suffering even worse fates.

There is also evidence that halogen sunlamps can cause the same bad effects as too much sun. So it doesn't help to get your tan in a tanning booth.

ACS Guidelines   The American Cancer Society offers these guidelines for preventing melanoma and other skin cancers: (1) always use a sunscreen, (2) wear protective clothing and a broad-brimmed hat,

(3) be extra careful during the sun's peak hours, (4) remember that clouds and haze do not completely block ultraviolet rays, and (5) reapply your sunscreen after long periods of swimming or sports activity.

50

AVOID

OCCUPATIONAL

EXPOSURES

Industrial Hazards A number of substances used in industry have been identified as cancer-causing agents.

Industrial processes and occupational exposures Be aware of these connections:

- Auramine manufacture—bladder
- Boot and shoe manufacture and repair—bladder, nasal
- Furniture manufacture—nasal
- Isopropyl alcohol manufacture—sinus
- Nickel refining—nasal, lung
- Rubber industry—bladder, others
- Underground hemotyte mining (exposure to radon) —lung

Chemicals and groups of chemicals Here is a list of the known carcinogens, followed by the types of cancer they are known to cause:

- 4-aminophynl—bladder
- Arsenic and arsenic compounds—lung, skin
- Asbestos—stomach, lung (mesothelioma)
- Benzene—leukemia
- Benzidine—bladder
- Bis (chloromethyl) ether—lung
- Chromium—lung
- Mustard gas—lung
- 2-naphthylamine—bladder
- Soots, tars, and oils—skin, lung, and bladder
- Vinyl chloride—liver (angiosarcoma)[1]

Numerous other substances are still under investigation for carcinogenicity. Be aware of them and follow the safety rules set up by the Occupational Safety and Health Administration for the minimization of exposure to these substances. Take all the precautions against cancer that you can—wherever you may be.

[1] International Agency for Research on Cancer, *IARC Monograph on the Evaluation of the Carcinogenic Risk of Chemicals to Humans, Chemicals, Industrial Processes, and Industries Associated with Cancer in Humans, IARC Monographs* vols. 1–29, *IARC Monographs* supplement 4 (Lyon, France: IARC, 1982).

OTHER THINGS
YOU SHOULD DO

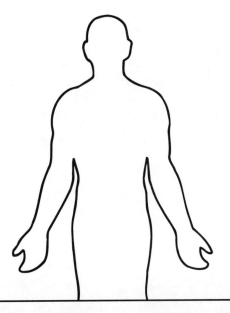

51

LAUGH
A LITTLE

In the Beginning In 1964, Norman Cousins fell dramatically ill with a rare and incurable disease that degenerates the collagen, or connective tissue, throughout the body. He checked himself out of the hospital and into a hotel. He played funny movies, read funny books, and did anything else he could think of to provoke laughter.

He initially intended to put himself into a positive frame of mind. But he quickly learned that laughter was also an antidote for the intense pain he'd been feeling: ten minutes of laughter would serve as a painkiller for two hours.

Cousins recovered and promptly began telling people about what had happened to him. The *New England Journal of Medicine* published an article he wrote, and he went on to write the best-selling book *Anatomy of an Illness as Perceived by the Patient.* The rest is history, for now laughter has become an integral part of the work of many cancer support groups, and some psychologists specialize in laughter-centered therapies.

Neurochemicals   Scientists now believe that a certain chemistry is associated with happiness and laughter. The physical link is apparently between chemicals manufactured in the brain (neurochemicals) and the body, including the immune system. When scientists finally unlock all the mysteries of these chemicals and the ways in which they interact with the rest of the human body, we may find another piece of the puzzle of preventing and possibly curing cancer. In the meantime, it's sufficient to know that laughter may be of value in fighting cancer. And even if it isn't, you've still enjoyed yourself. So have a good laugh. It can't hurt you, and it may actually help you.

52

SHARE
THIS BOOK
WITH
A FRIEND

Diet and Life-Style Changes   A panel of experts at the International Congress on Obesity set down some guidelines for the design of weight control programs. Some of the same principles apply to the prevention of cancer, for many of the things you can do to protect yourself against cancer involve diet and life-style changes just as does a reputable long-term weight loss program.

Indeed, to prevent cancer, you should achieve and then maintain your ideal weight, as we discussed earlier. An element of a good weight loss program is psychosocial support. The same is true of any major diet or life-style change, such as an anticancer program. Thus, your friends and family can play a very important role in helping you to do many of the things that will help prevent cancer.

Spread the News   One way to involve them is to share this book with them. If they understand some of the many reasons why you are changing your diet and life-style, they may be willing to help you achieve your goals. They may even be willing to join you. It is much easier to stay on a diet or engage in an exercise program if you have someone to do it with, especially if that someone is special to you.

In addition, you'll be helping to inform them about how to protect themselves against cancer. And then they may teach someone else and so on until you've started a whole chain of people who are practicing cancer prevention.

So share this book with a friend. If we all work together, we will eventually conquer this terrible plague we call cancer, and in the process we will learn some things that will keep us all generally healthier and happier.